Affordable
Anti Inflammatory
Recipe Book

Tasty and Delicious Vegetables and
Soup Recipes to Boost your Health

Mya Castillo

Table of Contents

Baked Avocado

Prep Time:
10 minutes
Cook Time:
20 minutes
Serve: 4

Ingredients:

- 2 avocados, peeled, pitted, halved
- 1 tablespoon olive oil
- ½ teaspoon dried thyme

Directions:

1.Put the avocado halves in the baking tray and sprinkle with olive oil and dried thyme.

2.Bake the avocados at 365F for 120 minutes.

Nutrition: 235 calories, 1.9g protein, 8.7g carbohydrates, 23.1g fat, 6.8g fiber, 0mg cholesterol, 6mg sodium, 488mg potassium

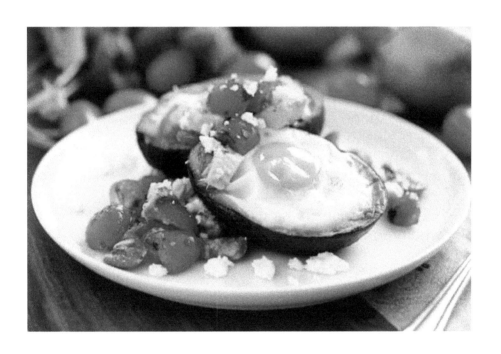

Baked Cremini Mushrooms

Prep Time:
10 minutes
Cook Time:
30 minutes
Serve: 4

Ingredients:

- 3 cups cremini mushrooms
- ¼ cup plain yogurt
- ¼ cup fresh parsley, chopped
- 1 teaspoon minced garlic
- 1 teaspoon ground turmeric
- 1 tablespoon olive oil

Directions:

1.Mix cremini mushrooms with plain yogurt, parsley, and all remaining ingredients.

2.Put the mixture in the tray and bake at 350F for 30 minutes.

Nutrition: 60 calories, 2.4g protein, 4.1g carbohydrates, 3.8g fat, 0.6g fiber, 1mg cholesterol, 16mg sodium, 315mg potassium

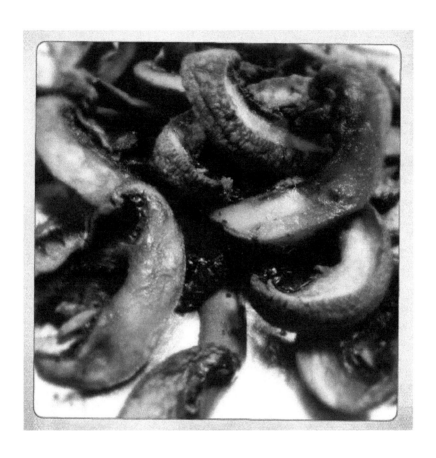

Bean Spread

Prep Time:
10 minutes
Cook Time:
0 minutes
Serve: 6

Ingredients:

- 2 cups red kidney beans, boiled
- 3 tablespoons plain yogurt
- 1 teaspoon ground nutmeg
- 1 teaspoon cayenne pepper
- 1 tablespoon fresh cilantro, chopped

Directions:

1.Blend the red kidney beans until you get a smooth paste.

2.Then mix the beans with plain yogurt, ground nutmeg, cayenne pepper, and cilantro.

3.Carefully mix the spread.

Nutrition: 215 calories, 14.3g protein, 38.5g carbohydrates, 0.9g fat, 9.5g fiber, 0mg cholesterol, 13mg sodium, 860mg potassium

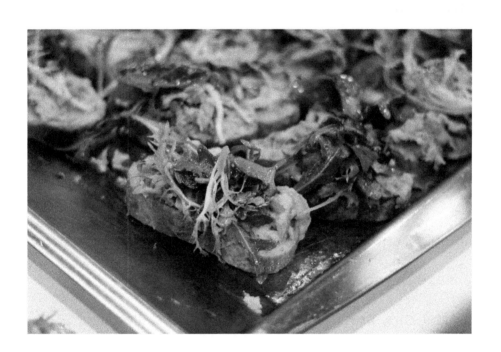

Eggplant Balls

Prep Time:
10 minutes
Cook Time:
5 minutes
Serve: 6

Ingredients:

- 2 cups eggplants, peeled, boiled
- ½ cup almond flour
- 1 teaspoon ground cumin
- ½ teaspoon ground coriander
- 1 teaspoon chili powder
- 1 tablespoon olive oil

Directions:

1.Blend the eggplant until smooth and mix it with almond flour, ground cumin, ground coriander, and chili powder.

2.Make the small balls.

3.After this, preheat the olive oil in the skillet well.

4.Put the eggplant balls inside and roast them for 2 minutes per side.

Nutrition: 86 calories, 2.4g protein, 4g carbohydrates, 7g fat, 2.2g fiber, 0mg cholesterol, 9mg sodium, 77mg potassium

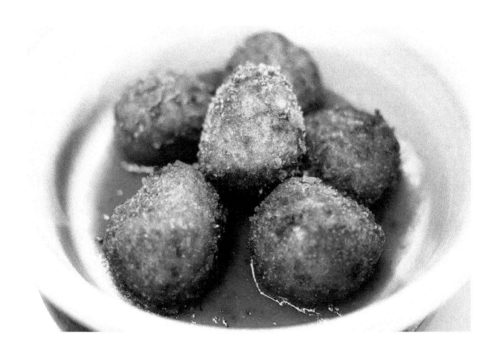

Spicy Artichoke

Prep Time:
10 minutes
Cook Time:
35 minutes
Serve: 2

Ingredients:

- 2 artichokes, halved
- 1 teaspoon minced garlic
- ½ teaspoon ground coriander
- ¼ teaspoon dried thyme
- 1 teaspoon dried oregano
- 4 teaspoons olive oil

Directions:

1.Put the artichokes in the tray.

2.Then rub them with minced garlic, ground coriander, dried thyme, and oregano.

3.Sprinkle the artichokes with olive oil and cook them at 350F for 35 minutes.

Nutrition: 161 calories, 5.5g protein, 18.1g carbohydrates, 9.7g fat, 9.2g fiber, 0mg cholesterol, 153mg sodium, 619mg potassium

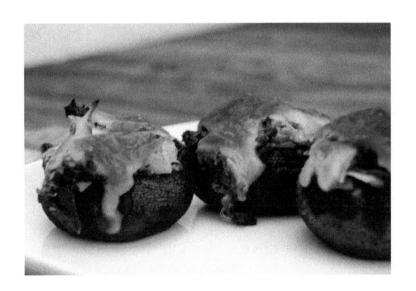

Mushrooms Cakes

Prep Time:
10 minutes
Cook Time:
10 minutes
Serve: 8

Ingredients:

- 3 cups mushrooms, sliced
- ½ cup almond flour
- 1 teaspoon chili flakes
- 1 teaspoon ground coriander
- 1 tablespoon olive oil
- ¼ cup plain yogurt

Directions:

1.In the mixing bowl, mix sliced mushrooms with almond flour, chili flakes, ground coriander, and yogurt.

2.Then preheat the olive oil well in the skillet.

3.Make the small cakes from the mushroom mixture and put in the hot skillet.

4.Roast the mushroom cakes for 4 minutes per side.

Nutrition: 68 calories, 2.8g protein, 2.9g carbohydrates, 5.3g fat, 1g fiber, 0mg cholesterol, 9mg sodium, 102mg potassium

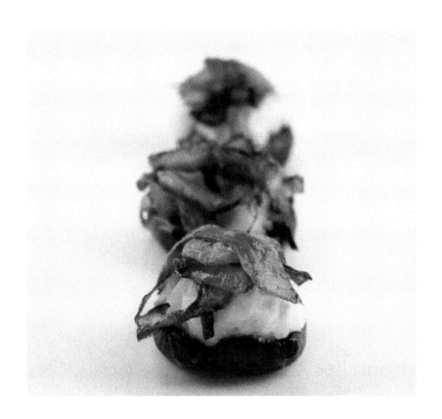

Baked Grapes

Prep Time:
10 minutes
Cook Time:
20 minutes
Serve: 6

Ingredients:

- 3 cups green grapes
- 1 oz raisins, chopped
- 1 tablespoon olive oil
- 1 tablespoon lemon juice
- 1 teaspoon dried oregano

Directions:

1.Mix grapes with raisins, olive oil, lemon juice, and dried oregano.

2.Put the mixture in the tray and bake at 360F for 20 minutes.

Nutrition: 66 calories, 0.5g protein, 11.8g carbohydrates, 2.6g fat, 0.7g fiber, 0mg cholesterol, 2mg sodium, 131mg potassium

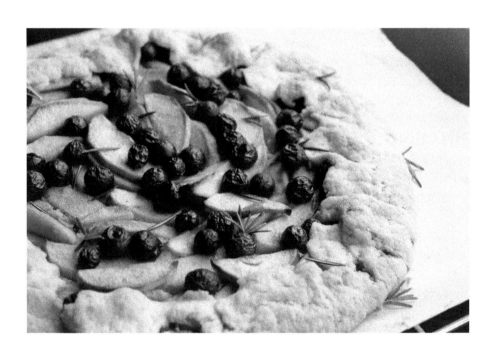

Green Peas Paste

Prep Time:
10 minutes
Cook Time:
0 minutes
Serve: 4

Ingredients:

- 2 cups green peas, boiled
- 1 tablespoon almond butter
- ¼ cup fresh parsley, chopped
- 2 tablespoons lemon juice

Directions:

1.Put all ingredients in the blender and blend until smooth.

2.Transfer the mixture into the serving bowl.

Nutrition: 86 calories, 5g protein, 11.6g carbohydrates, 2.6g fat, 4.3g fiber, 0mg cholesterol, 8mg sodium, 237mg potassium

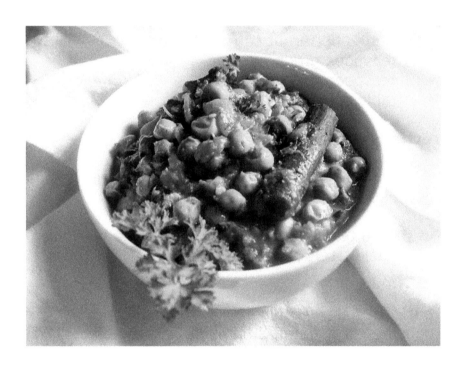

Baked Butternut Squash

Prep Time:
10 minutes
Cook Time:
35 minutes
Serve: 4

Ingredients:

- 1-pound butternut squash, chopped
- 1 teaspoon ground ginger
- 1 teaspoon ground paprika
- 1 tablespoon olive oil

Directions:

1.In the mixing bowl mix butternut squash with ground ginger, paprika, and olive oil.

2.Put the butternut squash mixture in the tray, flatten it well and bake at 360F for 35 minutes.

Nutrition: 84 calories, 1.3g protein, 13.9g carbohydrates, 3.7g fat, 2.5g fiber, 0mg cholesterol, 5mg sodium, 418mg potassium

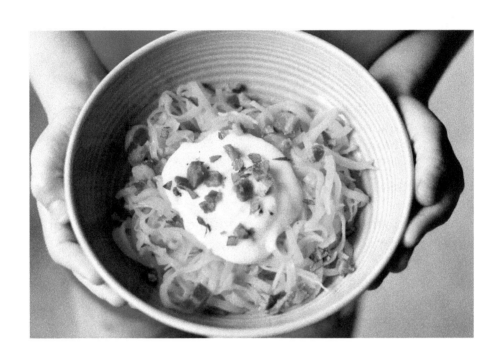

Cauliflower Balls

Prep Time:
10 minutes
Cook Time:
16 minutes
Serve: 4

Ingredients:

- 2 cups cauliflower, shredded
- 3 oz tofu, shredded
- 3 tablespoons almond flour
- 2 tablespoons coconut cream
- 1 teaspoon curry powder
- 1 tablespoon olive oil

Directions:

1.In the mixing bowl, mix shredded cauliflower with tofu, almond flour, coconut cream, and curry powder.

2.Make the balls from the mixture.

3.Then preheat the skillet well.

4.Add olive oil.

5.Then add cauliflower balls in the hot oil and roast them for 4 minutes per side or until the balls are light brown.

Nutrition: 108 calories, 4.1g protein, 4.9g carbohydrates, 8.8g fat, 2.3g fiber, 0mg cholesterol, 21mg sodium, 210mg potassium

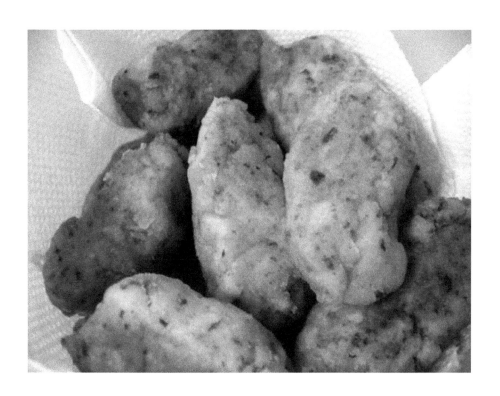

Baked Eggplants

Prep Time:
10 minutes
Cook Time:
30 minutes
Serve: 4

Ingredients:

- 4 eggplants, halved
- 1 teaspoon minced garlic
- 2 tablespoons olive oil

Directions:

1.Rub the eggplants with minced garlic and olive oil.

2.Put the eggplant halves in the tray and bake at 375F for 30 minutes.

Nutrition: 198 calories, 5.4g protein, 32.5g carbohydrates, 8g fat, 19.4g fiber, 0mg cholesterol, 11mg sodium, 1258mg potassium

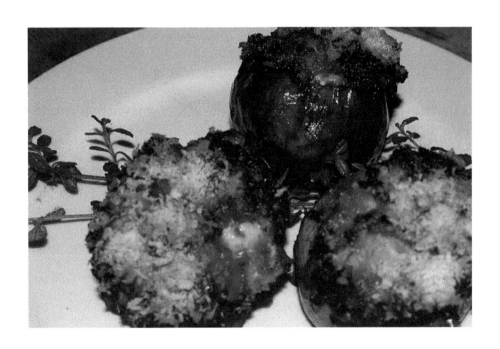

Zucchini Cakes

Prep Time:
10 minutes
Cook Time:
15 minutes
Serve: 4

Ingredients:

- 2 zucchinis, grated
- 3 tablespoons almond flour
- 1 teaspoon ground coriander
- 1 tablespoon olive oil

1.In the mixing bowl, mix grated zucchini with almond flour and ground coriander.

2.Preheat the skillet and pour the olive oil inside.

3.Preheat the oil.

4.Then make the cakes from the zucchini mixture and put them in the hot oil.

5.Cook the zucchini cakes for 3-4 minutes per side.

Nutrition: 77 calories, 2.3g protein, 4.4g carbohydrates, 6.2g fat, 1.6g fiber, 0mg cholesterol, 12mg sodium, 257mg potassium

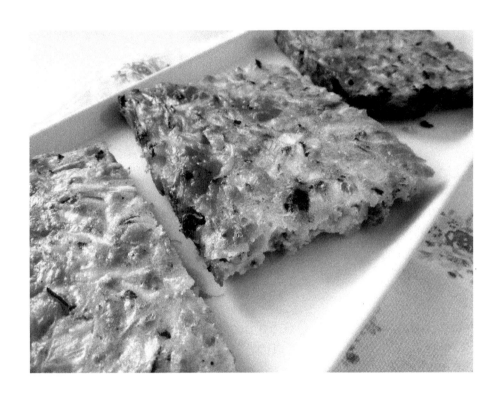

Baked Jalapenos

Prep Time:
10 minutes
Cook Time:
20 minutes
Serve: 4

Ingredients:

- 8 jalapenos, trimmed
- 1 tablespoon olive oil
- 1 teaspoon fennel seeds

Directions:

1.Line the baking tray with baking paper.

2.Then put the jalapenos in the baking tray and sprinkle with olive oil and fennel seeds.

3.Bake the jalapenos at 375F for 20 minutes.

Nutrition: 40 calories, 0.5g protein, 1.9g carbohydrates, 3.7g fat, 1g fiber, 0mg cholesterol, 1mg sodium, 69mg potassium

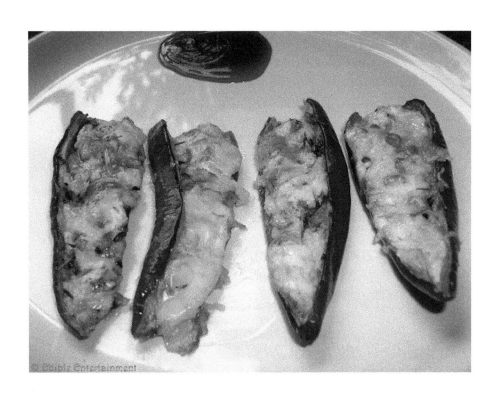

Baked Onions

Prep Time:
10 minutes
Cook Time:
20 minutes
Serve: 4

Ingredients:

- 4 red onions, peeled
- 1 teaspoon dried dill
- 1 teaspoon garlic powder
- 2 tablespoons olive oil

Directions:

1.Make the cuts in the onions and sprinkle them with dried dill, garlic powder, and olive oil.

2.Then wrap the onions in the foil and put in the tray.

3.Bake the onions at 400F for 20 minutes.

Nutrition: 107 calories, 1.4g protein, 10.9g carbohydrates, 7.1g fat, 2.5g fiber, 0mg cholesterol, 5mg sodium, 177mg potassium

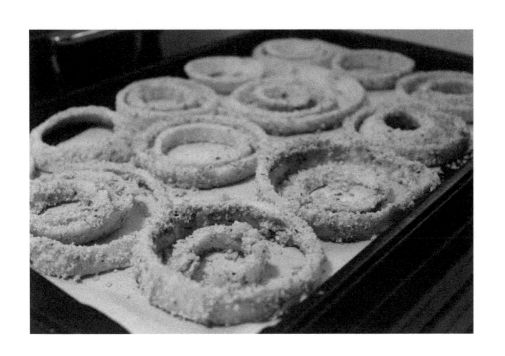

Mushroom Steaks

Prep Time:
10 minutes
Cook Time:
10 minutes
Serve: 2

Ingredients:

- 2 Portobello mushrooms
- 1 tablespoon olive oil
- ½ teaspoon ground black pepper

Directions:

1.Beat the mushrooms gently with the help of the kitchen hammer.

2.Then sprinkle the mushroom steaks with ground black pepper and olive oil.

3.Roast the mushrooms steaks in the well-preheat skillet for 5 minutes per side.

Nutrition: 81 calories, 3.1g protein, 3.3g carbohydrates, 7g fat, 1.1g fiber, 0mg cholesterol, 0mg sodium, 307mg potassium

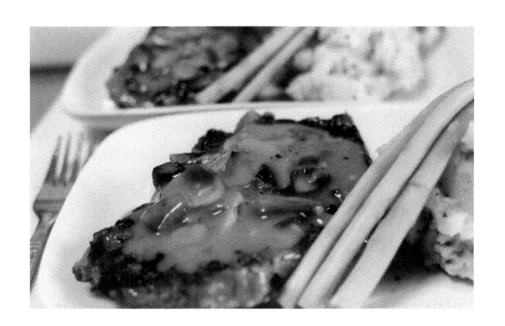

Baked Turnip

Prep Time:
10 minutes
Cook Time:
35 minutes
Serve: 3

Ingredients:

- 2 cups turnips, peeled, roughly chopped
- 1 tablespoon olive oil
- 1 teaspoon dried oregano

Directions:

1.Put the turnip in the baking tray and flatten it gently.

2.Sprinkle the vegetables with olive oil and dried oregano.

3.Bake the turnip at 355F for 35 minutes.

Nutrition: 65 calories, 0.7g protein, 5.7g carbohydrates, 4.7g fat, 1.5g fiber, 0mg cholesterol, 53mg sodium, 162mg potassium

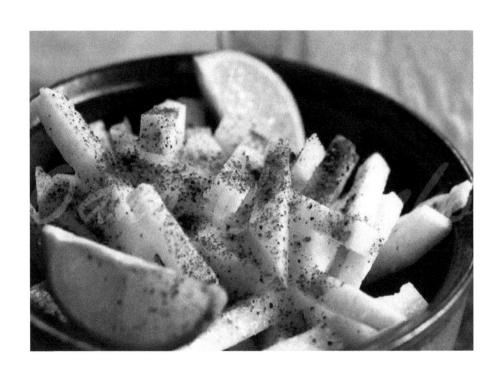

Avocado Spread

Prep Time:
10 minutes
Cook Time:
0 minutes
Serve: 2

Ingredients:

- 1 avocado, pitted, chopped, peeled
- ¼ cup plain yogurt
- 1 garlic clove, diced

Directions:

1.Put all ingredients in the blender and blend until smooth.

2.Transfer the spread in the serving bowl.

Nutrition: 229 calories, 3.8g protein, 11.3g carbohydrates, 20g fat, 6.8g fiber, 0mg cholesterol, 28mg sodium, 565mg potassium

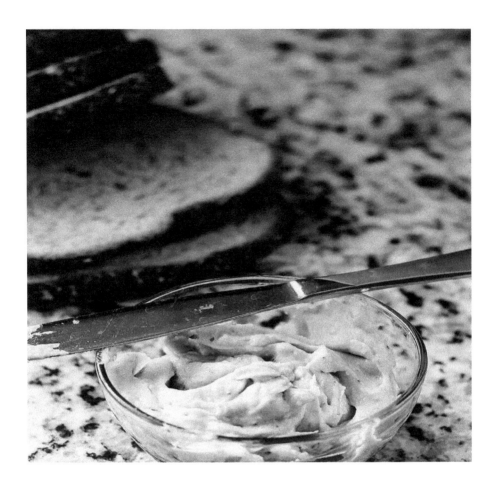

Burrito Bowl

Prep Time:
10 minutes
Cook Time:
0 minutes
Serve: 4

Ingredients:

- 4 tomatoes, chopped
- 1 cucumber, chopped
- ¼ cup quinoa, cooked
- 2 tablespoons plain yogurt
- 1 teaspoon ground coriander
- 1 teaspoon chili powder
- ¼ cup fresh cilantro, chopped

Directions:

1. Put all ingredients in the serving bowls and carefully mix them.

Nutrition: 81 calories, 3.7g protein, 15.4g carbohydrates, 1.2g fat, 2.9g fiber, 0mg cholesterol, 21mg sodium, 511mg potassium

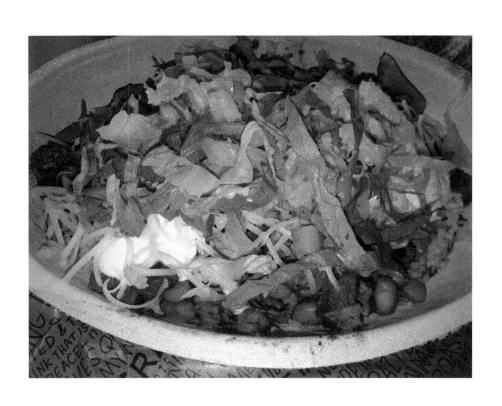

43

Grilled Peppers

Prep Time:
10 minutes
Cook Time:
8 minutes
Serve: 4

Ingredients:

- 4 sweet peppers
- 1 tablespoon olive oil
- 1 teaspoon fresh parsley, chopped
- 1 teaspoon sesame seeds

Directions:

1.Preheat the grill to 400F.

2.Put the sweet peppers in the grill and cook for 4 minutes per side.

3.Then peel the sweet peppers and chop them roughly.

4.Mix the chopped peppers with olive oil, parsley, and sesame seeds.

Nutrition: 72 calories, 1.3g protein, 9.2g carbohydrates, 4.2g fat, 1.7g fiber, 0mg cholesterol, 3mg sodium, 229mg potassium

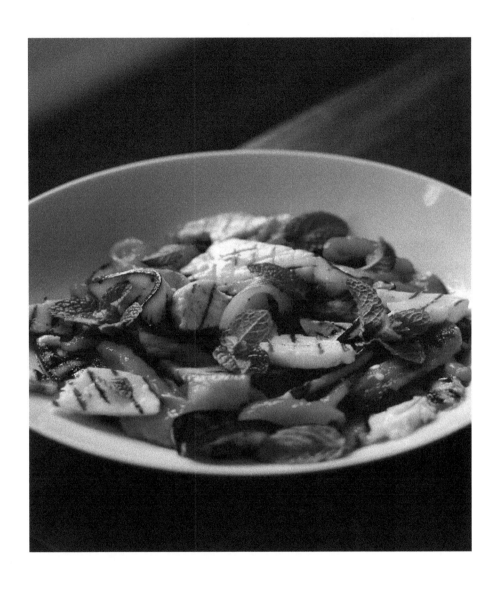

Parsley Guacamole

Prep Time:
10 minutes
Cook Time:
0 minutes
Serve: 4

Ingredients:

- 1 avocado, pitted, peeled and chopped
- ½ cup chopped parsley
- 2 lemons
- ¼ cup coconut cream

1.Mix avocado with parsley and coconut cream.

2.Gently blend the mixture.

3.Then squeeze the lemon juice in the avocado mixture.

4.Carefully mix the meal.

Nutrition: 148 calories, 1.8g protein, 8.3g carbohydrates, 13.5g fat, 4.8g fiber, 0mg cholesterol, 10mg sodium, 365mg potassium

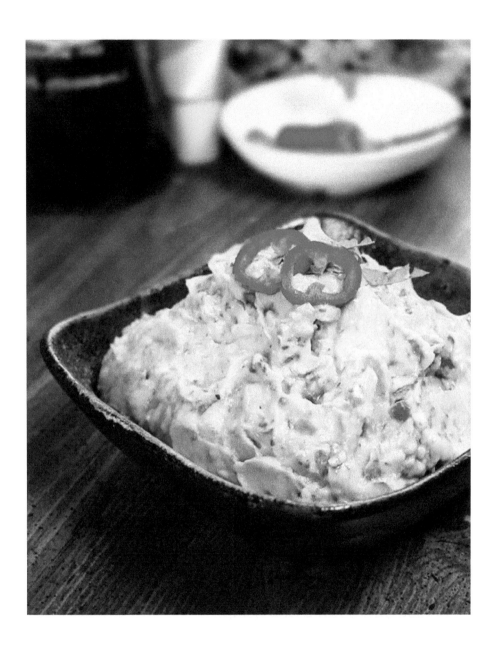

Baked Chickpeas

Prep Time:
10 minutes
Cook Time:
20 minutes
Serve: 4

Ingredients:

- 2 cups chickpeas, boiled
- 1 tablespoon olive oil
- 1 teaspoon chili powder
- 1 teaspoon ground black pepper
- 1 tablespoon dried oregano

Directions:

1.Line the baking tray with baking paper.

2.Then mix chickpeas with olive oil, chili powder, ground black pepper, and dried oregano.

3.Put the mixture in the baking tray and bake at 365F for 20 minutes.

Nutrition: 401 calories, 19.6g protein, 62.1g carbohydrates, 9.8g fat, 18.2g fiber, 0mg cholesterol, 31mg sodium, 913mg potassium

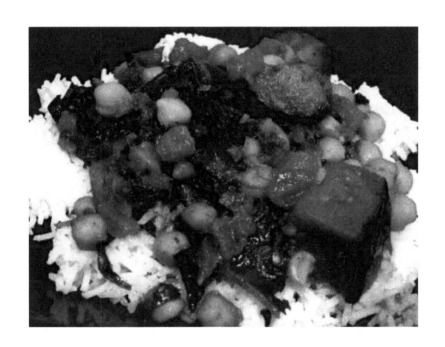

Broccoli Steaks

Prep Time:
10 minutes
Cook Time:
20 minutes
Serve: 4

Ingredients:

- 1-pound broccoli head
- 1 teaspoon cayenne pepper
- 2 tablespoons olive oil

Directions:

1.Slice the broccoli head into the steaks and put in the baking tray in one layer.

2.Sprinkle the vegetables with cayenne pepper and olive oil.

3.Bake the broccoli steaks at 365F for 10 minutes per side.

Nutrition: 100 calories, 3.2g protein, 7.8g carbohydrates, 7.5g fat, 3.1g fiber, 0mg cholesterol, 38mg sodium, 368mg potassium

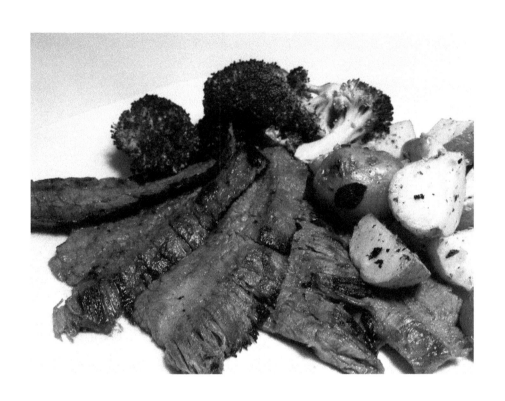

Lemon Bok Choy

Prep Time:
10 minutes
Cook Time:
20 minutes
Serve: 4

Ingredients:

- 1 pound bok choy, sliced
- 1 lemon
- 1 tablespoon olive oil
- 1 teaspoon cumin seeds

Directions:

1.Preheat the olive oil in the skillet well.

2.Add bok choy and roast it for 1 minute per side.

3.Then sprinkle the bok choy with cumin seeds.

4.Squeeze the lemon juice over the bok choy, carefully mix the meal, and cook it on low heat for 15 minutes.

Nutrition: 51 calories, 2g protein, 4.1g carbohydrates, 3.9g fat, 1.6g fiber, 0mg cholesterol, 75mg sodium, 315mg potassium

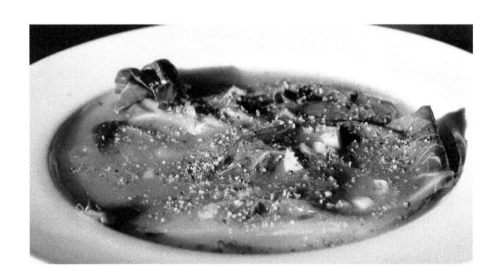

Tomato & Mushroom Soup

Prep Time:
55 Minutes
Serve: 4-6

Ingredients:

- 8Cups beef broth
- 1 Pound mushrooms (thin slices)
- 1 Garlic clove (minced)
- 6tbsp Butter
- 1 Can tomato sauce
- 2 Medium onions (chopped)
- 2 Medium tomatoes (peeled)
- 2 Chop carrots
- 2tbsp Salt &
- ½tbsp black pepper
- Sour cream
- 3tbsp fresh parsley
- 3 Celery ribs (chopped)
- 3tbsp All-purpose flour

Directions:

1.Sautee mushrooms with butter in a large kettle on medium flame.

2.In the same pot, Sautee carrots, garlic, onion, and celery with butter.

3.Now add beef broth, half mushrooms, tomato sauce, and tomato slices. Simmer it almost for15 minutes on medium flame.

4.Now add parsley with remaining mushrooms and stir for 15 minutes. Mix all-purpose flour in water and add it gradually in it.

5. Simmer for 10 minutes. Garnish it with sour cream.

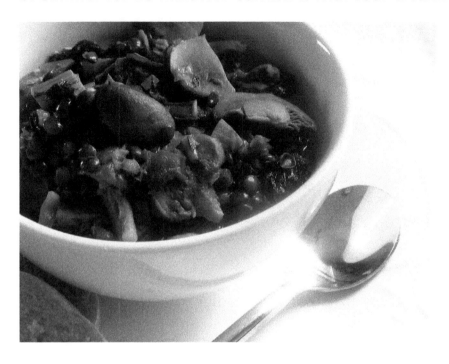

Broccoli & Cheese Soup

Prep Time:
40 Minutes
Serve: 4-5

Ingredients:

- 1 Medium onion (chopped)
- ½ Cup butter
- 14ounces Chicken Broth
- 1 Loaf cheese food (processed)
- 1tbsp Garlic Powder
- 3 Cans frozen broccoli
- 2/3 Cup corn starch
- 2 Cups milk
- 1 Cup water

Directions:

1.Melt butter in a pan on medium flame and cook the onion for 5 min.

2.In cooked onion add broccoli and chicken broth and stir for a few minutes.

3.Now add cheese cubes, garlic powder, and powder and cook it on low flame.

4.Mix cornstarch with water in a bowl and add it to the soup.

5.Simmer the soup for 15 minutes until all the cheese is melt.

6.Serve it hot with parsley and parmesan cheese.

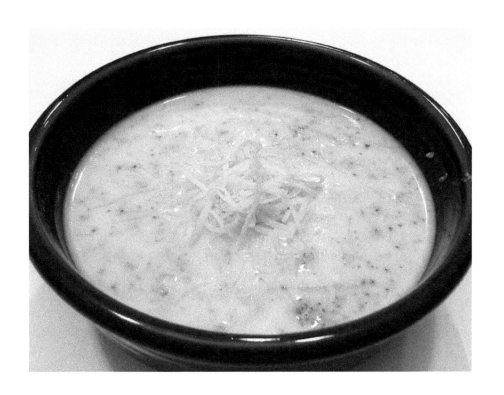

Creamy Chickpeas Stew

Prep Time:
15 minutes
Cook Time:
56 minutes
Serve: 4-6

Ingredients:

- ¼ cup coconut oil
- 1 medium yellow onion, chopped
- 2 teaspoons fresh ginger, chopped finely
- 2 minced garlic cloves
- 1 teaspoon ground cumin
- 1 teaspoon ground coriander
- ¾ teaspoon ground turmeric
- ¼ teaspoon yellow mustard seeds
- ¼ tsp cayenne pepper
- 1 (19-ounce) can chickpeas, rinsed and drained
- 2 large sweet potatoes, peeled and cubed into 1-inch size
- 1 pound fresh kale, trimmed and chopped
- 5 cups vegetable broth
- Salt, to taste
- 1 cup coconut milk
- ¼ cup red bell pepper, seeded and julienned
- 2 tablespoons fresh cilantro, chopped

Directions:

1.In a large pan, heat oil on medium heat.

2.Add onion and sauté for about 3 minutes.

3.Add ginger and garlic and sauté for about 2 minutes.

4.Add spices and sauté for about 1 minute.

5.Add chickpeas, sweet potato, kale and broth and bring to a boil on medium-high heat.

6.Reduce the heat to medium-low and simmer, covered for about 35 minutes.

7.Stir in coconut milk and simmer for about 15 minutes or till desired thickness of stew.

8.Serve hot with garnishing of bell pepper and cilantro.

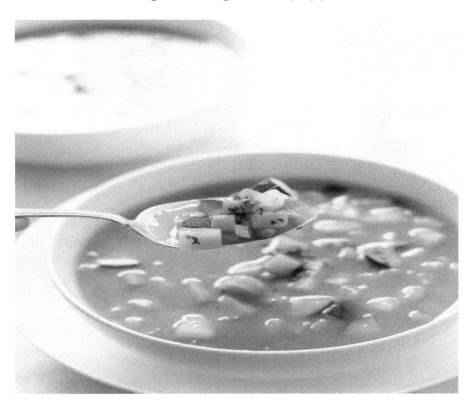

Lentil Stew

Prep Time:
15 minutes
Cook Time:
50 minutes
Serve: 4

Ingredients:

- 1 cup dry lentils, rinsed and drained
- 1 cup potato, peeled and chopped
- ½ cup celery, chopped
- ½ cup carrot, peeled and chopped
- ½ cup onion, chopped
- 1 garlic clove, minced
- 1 (14½-ounce) peeled Italian tomatoes, chopped
- 1 tablespoon dried basil, crushed
- 1 tablespoon dried parsley, crushed
- Freshly ground black pepper, to taste
- 3½ cups chicken broth

Directions:

1.In a large pan, add all ingredients and stir to combine.

2.Bring to a boil on high heat.

3.Reduce the heat to low and simmer, covered for about 45-50 minutes, stirring occasionally.

Nutrition: Calories: 261, Fat: 1g, Sat Fat: 5g, Carbohydrates: 43g, Fiber: 18g, Sugar: 2g, Protein: 19g, Sodium: 678mg

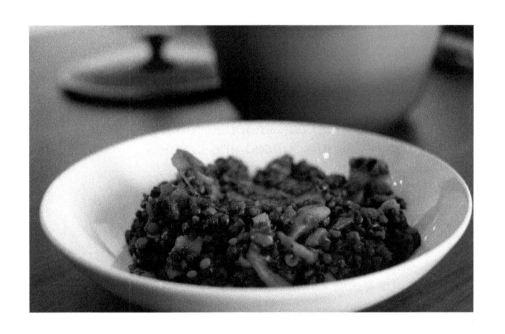

Lentil & Quinoa Stew

Prep Time:
15 minutes
Cook Time:
34 minutes
Serve: 4-6

Ingredients:

- 1 tablespoon coconut oil
- 3 carrots, peeled and chopped
- 3 celery stalks, chopped
- 1 yellow onion, chopped
- 4 garlic cloves, minced
- 1 (26½-ounce) can chopped tomatoes
- 1 cup red lentils, rinsed and drained
- ½ cup quinoa
- 1½ teaspoons ground cumin
- ½ teaspoon ground turmeric
- ½ teaspoon ground ginger
- Salt, to taste
- 5 cups water
- 2 cups fresh kale, chopped

Directions:

1.In a large pan, heat oil on medium heat.

2.Add celery, onion and carrot and sauté for about 8 minutes.

3.Add garlic and sauté for about 1 minute.

4.Add remaining ingredients except kale and bring to a boil.

5.Reduce the heat to low and simmer, covered for about 20 minutes.

6.Stir in kale and simmer for about 4-5 minutes.

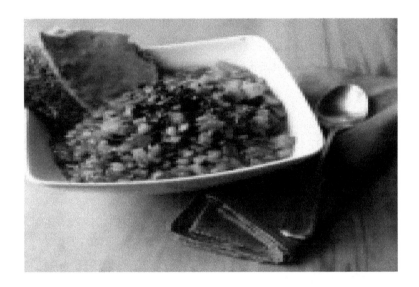

Chilled Tomato & Bell Pepper Soup

Prep Time:
25 minutes
Cook Time:
20 seconds
Serve: 4-6

Ingredients:

- 8 ripe Roma tomatoes
- 1 small red bell pepper, seeded and chopped roughly
- 1 small green bell pepper, seeded and chopped roughly
- 1 medium cucumber, peeled, seeded and chopped roughly
- 1 small red onion, chopped roughly
- 3 large garlic cloves, chopped
- 1 fresh long red chili, seeded and chopped roughly
- 2 teaspoons fresh orange zest, grated finely
- 1 cup fresh tomato juice
- ¾ cup olive oil
- 2-3 tablespoons fresh orange juice
- 2 tablespoons apple cider vinegar
- 1 cup chilled water
- 1 teaspoon salt
- ½ freshly ground black pepper

Directions:

1.In a large pan of boiling water, add tomatoes and boil for 20 seconds or till the skin begins to crack.

2.Drain well and rinse under cold water. Then peel the skin of tomatoes. Cut the tomatoes and discard the seeds.

3.In a large food processor, add tomatoes and keep all ingredients and pulse till smooth.

4.Refrigerate to chill for about 1 hour before serving.

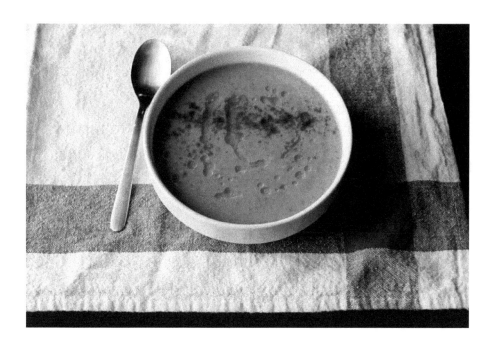

Chilled Peas Soup

Prep Time:
10 minutes
Cook Time:
20 seconds
Serve: 4

Ingredients:

- ½ tablespoons coconut oil
- 1 large shallot, minced
- 10 fresh mint leaves
- 2 cups homemade chicken broth
- 1 pound frozen baby peas
- Salt and freshly ground black pepper, to taste

Directions:

1.In a medium pan, heat oil on medium-high heat.

2.Add shallots and sauté for about 1 minute.

3.Add mint and broth and bring to a boil.

4.Stir in peas and again bring to a boil.

5.Reduce the heat to medium-low. Simmer for about 4 minutes.

6.Season with salt and black pepper and remove from heat. Let it cool slightly.

7.Transfer the soup in a blender and pulse till smooth.

8.Refrigerate to chill for about 1 hour before serving.

Nutrition: Calories: 119, fat: 9g, carbohydrates: 18g, sugar: 9g, protein: 7g, fiber: 7g

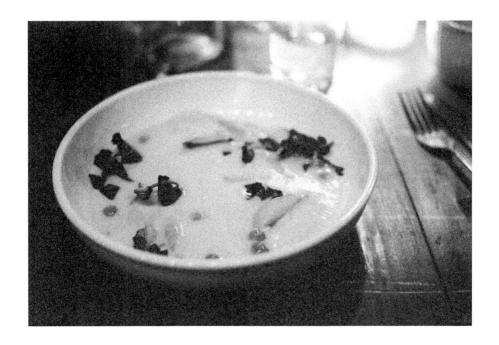

Chilled Spinach & Cucumber Soup

Prep Time:
15 minutes
Serve: 2

Ingredients:

- 2 medium cucumbers, peeled seeded and chopped
- 2 cups fresh spinach
- 1 small avocado, peeled, pitted and chopped
- ½ of jalapeño, seeded and chopped
- 1cup mixed fresh herbs
- 1 cup water
- 1 tablespoon fresh lime juice
- 1 tablespoon olive oil

Directions:

1.In a large food processor, add all ingredients and pulse till smooth.

2.Refrigerate to chill for about 2 hours before serving.

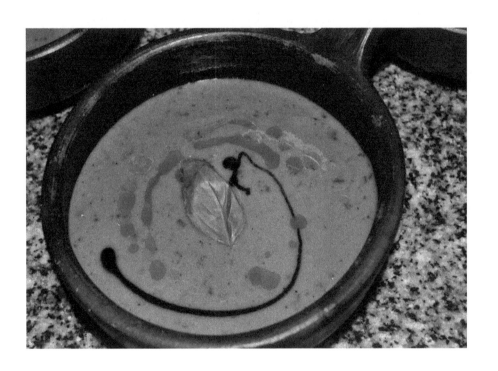

Chilled Fruit Soup

Prep Time:
15 minutes
Serve: 4

Ingredients:

For Soup:

- 2 pounds fresh strawberries, hulled and sliced
- ½ of medium watermelon, seeded and chopped

For Raspberry Sauce:

- 6-ounce fresh raspberries
- ¼ cup coconut milk
- 1 teaspoon fresh lemon zest, grated finely
- 1 tablespoon fresh lemon juice

Directions:

1.In a bowl, add watermelon and strawberries. With a hand blender, blend till a smooth and creamy mixture forms.

2.Refrigerate to chill.

3.In a bowl, add raspberries and mash with a fork completely.

4.Add remaining ingredients and stir to combine well. Refrigerate to chill.

5.Divide the soup in serving bowls. Top with raspberry sauce and serve.

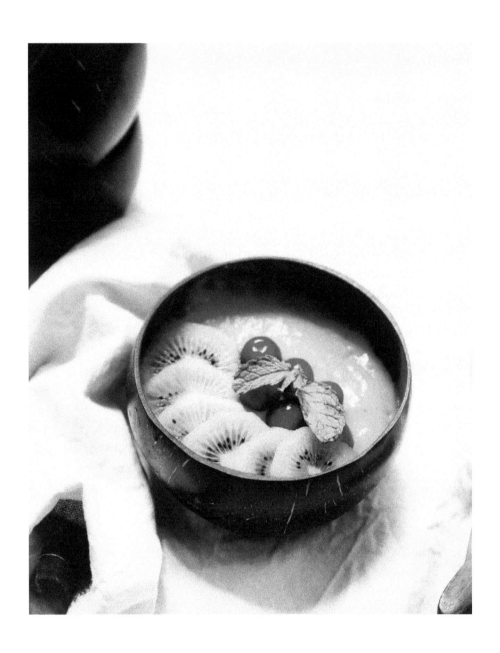

Chilled Pineapple Soup

Prep Time:
15 minutes
Serve: 4

Ingredients:

- 1 under ripe pineapple, peeled, cored and chopped
- ½ cup cucumber, peeled, seeded and chopped finely
- ½ cup red bell pepper, seeded and chopped finely
- ¼ cup red onion, chopped finely
- 1 tablespoon fresh cilantro, chopped finely
- ¼ of serrano Chile, seeded and minced
- 2 tablespoons fresh lime juice
- ½ teaspoon salt

Directions:

1.In a blender, add pineapple and pulse till pureed.

2.Strain the puree in a bowl.

3.Stir in remaining ingredients. Cover and chill for about 2 hours before serving.

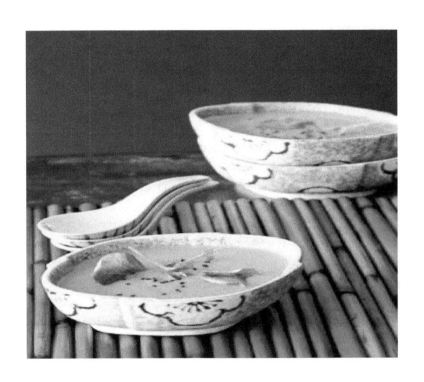

Creamy Cauliflower Soup

Prep Time:
15 minutes
Cook Time: 22-25 minutes
Serve: 4-6

Ingredients:

- 1 tablespoon extra-virgin olive oil
- 1 medium onion, chopped
- 4 garlic cloves, minced
- Salt, to taste
- 1 medium head cauliflower, cut into 1-inch pieces
- 4 ½-5½ cups water
- 1 avocado, peeled, pitted and chopped
- 2-3 cups mixed greens
- Freshly ground black pepper, to taste
- Fresh chopped parsley, for garnishing

Directions:

1.In a large soup pan, heat oil on medium heat.

2.Add onion and sauté for about 4-5 minutes.

3.Add garlic and pinch of salt and sauté for about 2-3 minutes.

4.Stir in cauliflower and ad water. Bring to a boil on high heat.

5.Reduce the heat to low. Simmer for about 10 minutes.

6.Stir in avocado and greens and simmer for about 3 minutes.

7.Remove from heat and cool slightly.

8.In a blender, transfer the soup in batches and pulse till smooth.

9.Add the soup in the pan on medium heat. Cook for about 3-4 minutes.

10.Stir in salt and black pepper and remove from heat.

11.Serve with the garnishing of parsley.

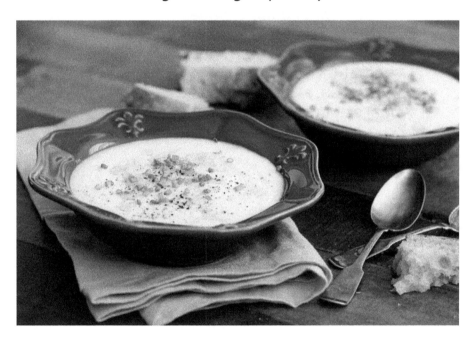

Creamy Carrot Soup

Prep Time:
15 minutes
Cook Time:
25 minutes
Serve: 2-3

Ingredients:

- 3 cups homemade vegetable broth
- 1½ cups fennel bulb, chopped
- 3 cups carrots, peeled and chopped
- 2 garlic cloves, minced
- 1 cup full-fat coconut milk
- Salt, to taste
- 4-ounces pancetta, chopped
- ½ cup pine nuts, toasted and chopped

Directions:

1.In a large soup pan, add broth and vegetables and a boil on high heat.

2.Reduce the heat to medium-low. Simmer for about 15-20 minutes.

3.Stir in coconut milk and simmer for about 3-5 minutes. Stir in salt and remove from heat.

4.Meanwhile heat a nonstick skillet on medium-high heat.

5.Add pancetta and cook for about 8-10 minutes or till crispy.

6.Serve this soup hot with the topping of cooked pancetta and pine nuts.

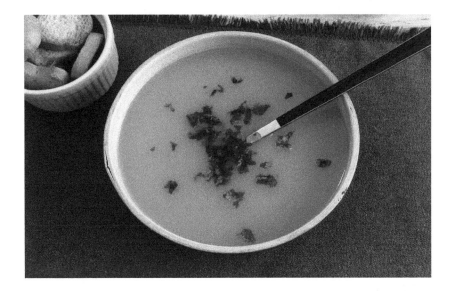

Green Veggie Soup

Prep Time:
20 minutes
Cook Time:
25 minutes
Serve: 6

Ingredients:

- 2 tablespoons ghee (clarified butter)
- 3-4 garlic cloves, minced
- 4 leeks (white part), chopped roughly
- 2 medium heads broccoli, chopped roughly
- ½ of small head cauliflower, chopped roughly
- 4 celery sticks, chopped roughly
- 8 cups homemade vegetable broth
- 2-3 cups fresh baby spinach
- 1 cup fresh parsley, chopped
- Freshly ground black pepper, to taste
- Pinch of ground nutmeg
- 1 tablespoon coconut cream

Directions:

1.In a large soup pan, heat oil on medium heat.

2.Add garlic and leeks and sauté for about 4-5 minutes.

3.Add broccoli, cauliflower and celery and sauté for about 5 minutes.

4.Add broth and bring to a boil. Reduce the heat to low. Simmer for about 10-15 minutes.

5.Stir in spinach and parsley and remove from heat.

6.With an immense blender, blend till pureed. Stir in nutmeg and black pepper.

7.Top with the dollop of coconut cream and serve.

Nutrition: Calories: 108, fat: 3g, carbohydrates: 17g, protein: 7g, fiber: 6g

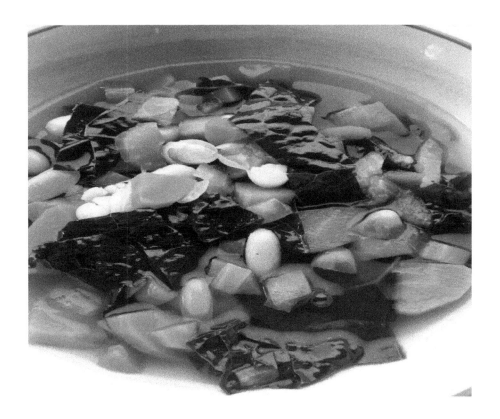

Chicken & Veggie Soup

Prep Time:
20 minutes
Cook Time:
28-30 minutes
Serve: 4

Ingredients:

- 2 tablespoons coconut oil
- 1 bunch scallion, sliced thinly
- 2-inch piece fresh ginger, minced
- 4 garlic cloves, minced
- 1 cup shiitake mushrooms, sliced
- 1 large carrot, peeled and shredded
- 1 red bell pepper, seeded and chopped
- 1 jalapeño pepper, chopped
- 14-ounces coconut milk
- 4 cups chicken broth
- 1 tablespoon red bat fish sauce
- 1 pound skinless, boneless chicken breasts Fresh cilantro, as required
- 1 teaspoon fresh lime zest, grated finely
- Salt and freshly ground black pepper, to taste

Directions:

1.In a large soup pan, heat oil on medium heat.

2.Add scallion, ginger and garlic and sauté for about 2-3 minutes.

3.Add mushrooms, carrot, bell pepper and jalapeño pepper and sauté for about 5 minutes.

4.Add broth, coconut milk, fish sauce and chicken and bring to a boil.

5.Reduce the heat to low. Simmer for about 15 minutes.

6.Transfer the chicken into a plate and chop into small chunks.

7.Add chopped chicken, cilantro, lime zest, salt and black pepper and simmer for 5 minutes more.

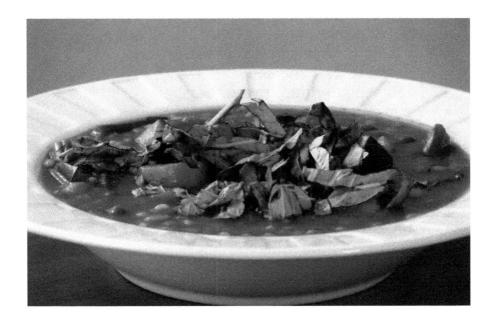

Mushroom Soup

Prep Time:
20 minutes
Cook Time:
30 minutes
Serve: 4

Ingredients:

- ½-ounce dried porcini mushrooms
- 2 tablespoons ghee (clarified butter)
- 1 celery stalk, chopped
- 1 large leek (pale part), chopped
- 1 small sweet potato, peeled and chopped
- 15 medium crimini mushrooms, sliced roughly
- 3 garlic cloves, minced
- 1 tablespoon dried thyme, crushed
- 3 cups homemade chicken broth
- ½ teaspoon Dijon mustard
- 1 tablespoon red boat fish sauce
- 2 bay leaves
- 1 teaspoon fresh lemon zest, grated finely
- ½ teaspoon freshly ground black pepper
- 3 tablespoons almond butter
- 1 tablespoon fresh lemon juice

Directions:

1.In a bowl, soak porcini mushrooms in boiling water. Keep aside for about 15-20 minutes.

2.Strain the mushrooms, reserving ½ cup of liquid. Then chop the mushrooms.

3.In a large soup pan, heat ghee on medium heat.

4.Add celery and leek and sauté for about 5-7 minutes.

5.Add sweet potato, cremini mushrooms, garlic and thyme and sauté for about 1-2 minutes.

6.Add broth, mustard, fish sauce, bay leaves, lemon zest, black pepper and cremini mushrooms with reserved liquid and bring to a boil.

7.Reduce the heat to low. Cover and simmer for about 15 minutes.

8.Uncover and simmer for 5 minutes more.

9.Stir in almond butter and lemon juice and serve hot.

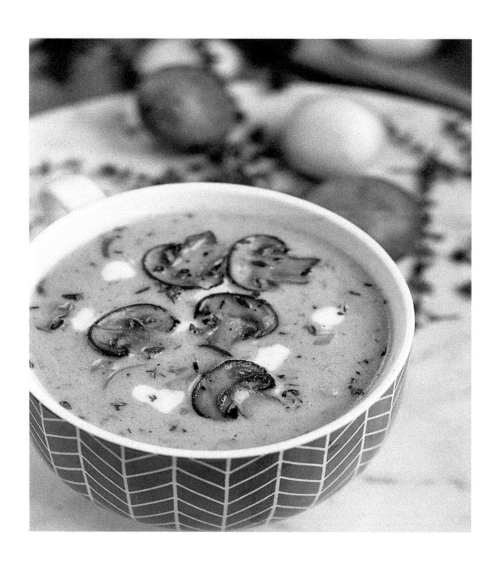

Roasted Veggies Soup

Prep Time:
20 minutes
Cook Time:
30 minutes
Serve: 4-6

Ingredients:

- 2½ pounds zucchini, cut into 1-inch pieces
- ½ of yellow onion, chopped
- 1 leek, chopped
- 3 garlic cloves, peeled
- 2 tablespoons coconut oil, melted
- 2½ cups water
- ½ cup raw cashews, soaked for 3 hours
- Salt and freshly ground black pepper, to taste

Directions:

1.Preheat the oven to 400 degrees F. Line a baking sheet with a parchment paper.

2.Arrange zucchini, onion, leek and garlic onto prepared baking sheet.

3.Roast for about 20 minutes. Remove from oven and cool slightly.

4.In a blender, add roasted veggies, water and cashews and pulse till smooth.

5.Transfer the pureed mixture in a soup pan on medium heat.

6.Simmer for about 5 minutes. Stir in salt and black pepper and remove from heat.

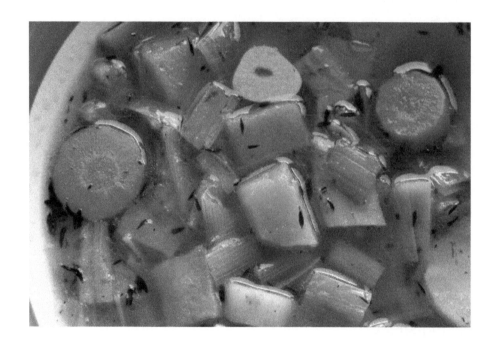

Chicken & Asparagus Soup

Prep Time:
20 minutes
Cook Time:
20 minutes
Serve: 8

Ingredients:

- 1 tablespoon coconut oil
- 1 onion, chopped
- 2 cups mushrooms, sliced thinly
- 1 celery stalk, chopped
- 2 cups grass-fed boneless chicken, chopped
- 15-20 fresh asparagus spears, trimmed and chopped
- 6-8 cups homemade chicken broth
- 14-ounce coconut milk
- 2 cups fresh spinach, chopped
- Salt and freshly ground black pepper, to taste

Directions:

1.In a large soup pan, heat oil on medium heat.

2.Add onion, mushrooms and celery and sauté for about 5 minutes.

3.Add chicken, asparagus and broth and bring to a boil.

4.Reduce the heat to low. Simmer for about 10 minutes.

5.Stir in coconut milk and spinach and bring to a boil on high heat.

6.Reduce the heat to low. Simmer for about 3-4 minutes.

7.Stir in salt and black pepper and remove from heat.

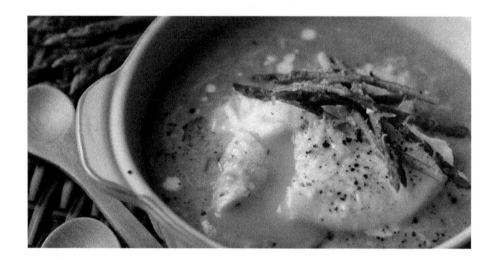

Shrimp & Snow Peas Soup

Prep Time:
15 minutes
Cook Time:
8-10 minutes
 Serve: 8

Ingredients:

- 4 teaspoons coconut oil
- 4 medium scallions (white and green part), sliced thinly
- 2-inch piece fresh ginger root, sliced thinly
- 8 cups homemade chicken broth
- ¼ teaspoon red boat fish sauce
- ¼ cup coconut aminos
- 1/8 teaspoon freshly ground white pepper
- 1 pound shrimp, peeled and deveined
- 1 (5-ounce) can sliced bamboo shoots, drained
- ½ pound snow peas, cleaned
- 1 tablespoon sesame oil, toasted

Directions:

1.In a large soup pan, heat oil on medium heat.

2.Add white part of scallion and ginger and sauté for about 2 minutes.

3.Add broth, fish sauce, coconut aminos and white pepper and bring to a boil.

4.Stir in shrimp, bamboo shoots and snow peas.

5.Reduce the heat to low. Simmer for about 2-3 minutes.

6.Stir in sesame oil and green part of scallion and remove from heat.

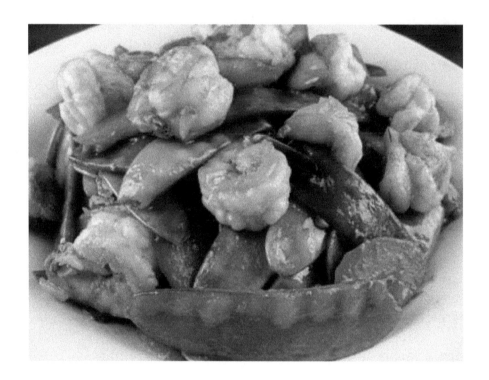

Zucchini & Squash Soup

Prep Time:
15 minutes
Cook Time:
12-15 minutes
Serve: 4

Ingredients:

- 2 tablespoons coconut oil
- 1 small onion, chopped
- 3 garlic cloves, minced
- 1 teaspoon ground cumin
- 1½ pounds yellow squash, chopped
- 3 cups zucchini, chopped
- 2 tablespoons jalapeño peppers, chopped finely
- 4 cups homemade vegetable broth
- 1 cup coconut milk
- 3 tablespoons fresh lemon juice
- ¼ cup fresh cilantro, chopped
- 2 tablespoons nutritional yeast
- Avocado slices, for garnishing

Directions:

1.In a large soup pan, heat oil on medium heat.

2.Add onion and sauté for about 4-5 minutes.

3.Add garlic and cumin and sauté for about 1 minute.

4.Add squash and zucchini and sauté for about 3-4 minutes.

5.Add jalapeño peppers and broth and bring to a boil. Immediately, turn off the heat.

91

6.Keep, covered for about 10 minutes.

7.Stir in coconut milk, lemon juice, cilantro and nutritional yeast and again bring to a boil.

8.Serve hot with the topping of avocado slices.

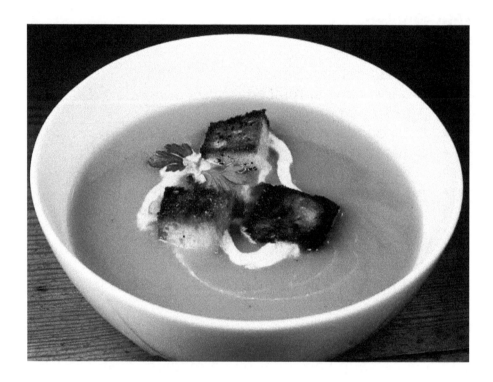

Spicy Leek Soup With Poached Eggs

Prep Time:
15 minutes
Cook Time:
10 minutes
Serve: 6-8

Ingredients:

- 2 tablespoons coconut oil
- 1 large leek, sliced
- 4 carrots, peeled and sliced
- 6 garlic cloves, minced
- 6-8 cups chicken broth
- ¾ teaspoon dried oregano, crushed
- ½ teaspoon paprika
- Pinch of red pepper flakes, crushed
- 2 teaspoons unrefined salt
- 6-8 organic eggs

Directions:

1.In a large soup pan, heat oil on medium heat.

2.Add leeks and sauté for about 3-4 minutes.

3.Add carrots and cook for about 4-5 minutes.

4.Add garlic and sauté for about 1 minute.

5.Add broth, oregano and spices and bring to a boil. Reduce the heat to low.

6.Simmer for about 1o minutes.

7.Meanwhile in a frying pan, add 1-2-inch water and bring to a gentle simmer. Stir in some salt.

8.Carefully, crack eggs in pan and cook for about 3-4 minutes on medium-low heat.

9.With a slotted spoon, place 1 egg in each bowl.

10. Divide the soup in bowls evenly and serve.

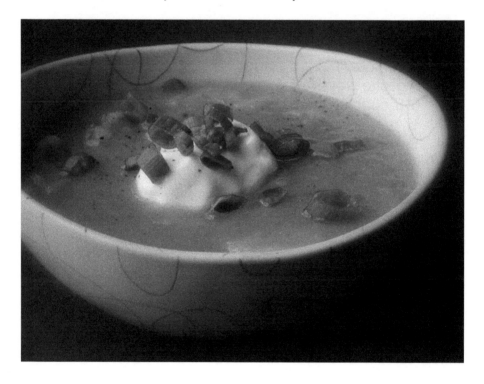

Parmesan Kale

Prep Time:
5 minutes
Cook Time:
20 minutes
Serve: 4

Ingredients:

- 4 cups kale, roughly chopped
- 2 oz Parmesan, grated
- 1 tablespoon olive oil

Directions:

1.Put the kale in the tray and flatten it well.

2.Then sprinkle the kale with olive oil and Parmesan.

3.Cook the kale at 350F for 20 minutes.

Nutrition: 109 calories, 6.6g protein, 7.5g carbohydrates, 6.5g fat, 1g fiber, 10mg cholesterol, 161mg sodium, 329mg potassium

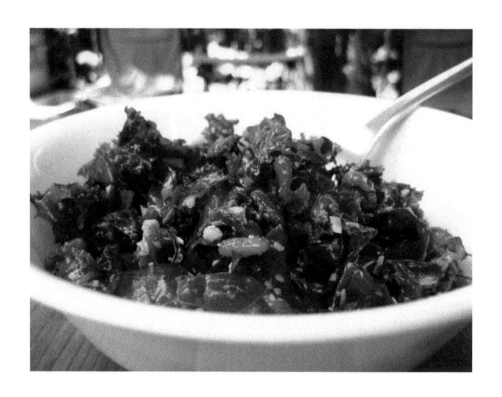

Curry Tofu

Prep Time:
20 minutes
Cook Time:
5 minutes
Serve: 4

Ingredients:

- 1-pound tofu, cubed
- 1 teaspoon curry powder
- 1 tablespoon olive oil
- ½ cup coconut cream
- 1 teaspoon lemon zest, grated

Directions:

1.In the mixing bowl, mix curry powder with olive oil, coconut cream, and lemon zest.

2.Then add tofu and mix well.

3.Leave the mixture for 10 minutes to marinate.

4.Then preheat the skillet well.

5.Add tofu and cook it for 2 minutes per side.

Nutrition: 180 calories, 10.1g protein, 4g carbohydrates, 15.5g fat, 1.9g fiber, 0mg cholesterol, 18mg sodium, 256mg potassium

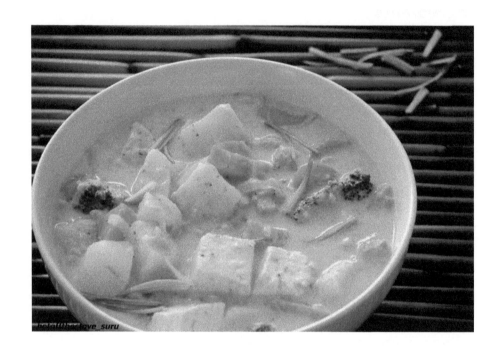

Cumin Zucchini Rings

Prep Time:
10 minutes
Cook Time:
15 minutes
Serve: 5

Ingredients:

- 3 zucchinis, sliced
- 1 tablespoon cumin seeds
- 1 tablespoon olive oil
- ¼ teaspoon cayenne pepper

Directions:

1.Line the baking tray with baking paper.

2.Put the zucchini slices inside the baking tray in one layer.

3.Then sprinkle them with cumin seeds, olive oil, and cayenne pepper.

4.Bake the zucchini rings for 15 minutes at 360F.

Nutrition: 48 calories, 1.6g protein, 4.5g carbohydrates, 3.3g fat, 1.4g fiber, 0mg cholesterol, 14mg sodium, 331mg potassium

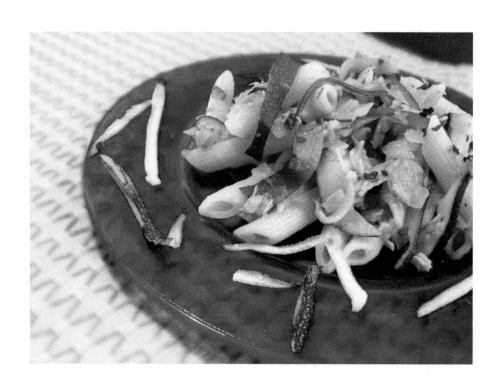

Chickpeas Spread

Prep Time:
10 minutes
Cook Time:
0 minutes
Serve: 3

Ingredients:

- 1 cup chickpeas, cooked
- 1 tablespoon tahini paste
- 2 tablespoons lemon juice
- ¼ cup olive oil

Directions:

1.Put all ingredients in the blender.

2.Blend the mixture until smooth.

3.Transfer it in the serving bowl.

Nutrition: 419 calories, 13.8g protein, 41.7g carbohydrates, 23.6g fat, 12.1g fiber, 0mg cholesterol, 24mg sodium, 617mg potassium

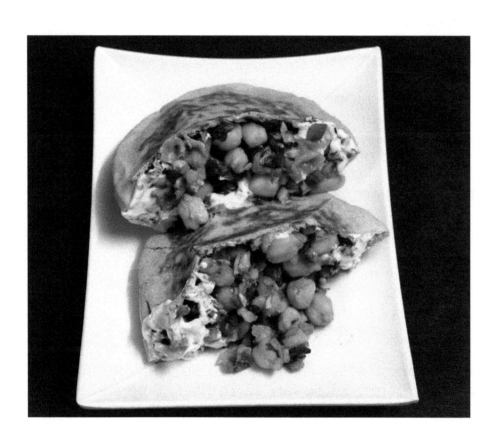

Mushroom Caps

Prep Time:
10 minutes
Cook Time:
20 minutes
 Serve: 5

Ingredients:

- 5 Portobello mushrooms (caps)
- 3 oz tofu, shredded
- ½ teaspoon curry paste
- 2 tablespoons coconut cream
- 1 teaspoon olive oil

Directions:

1.In the mixing bowl, mix curry powder with coconut cream, olive oil, and shredded tofu.

2.Then fill the mushrooms with the shredded tofu mixture and put in the tray in one layer.

3.Bake the mushrooms at 360F for 20 minutes.

Nutrition: 57 calories, 4.6g protein, 3.8g carbohydrates, 3.4g fat, 1.3g fiber, 0mg cholesterol, 3mg sodium, 341mg potassium

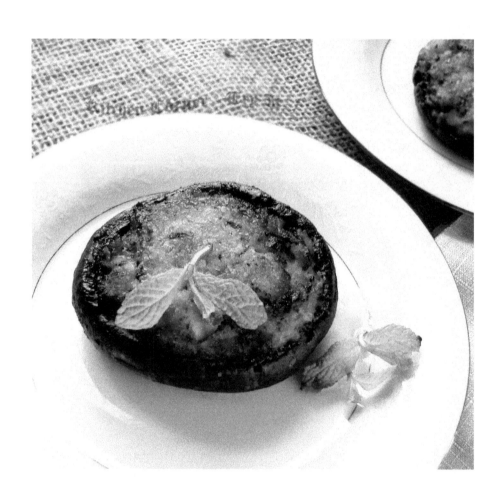

Ginger Baked Mango

Prep Time:
10 minutes
Cook Time:
20 minutes
Serve: 4

Ingredients:

- 2 mangos, pitted, halved
- 1 teaspoon minced ginger
- 1 tablespoon olive oil
- ¼ teaspoon dried rosemary

Directions:

1.Put the mango halves in the baking tray and sprinkle with olive oil.

2.Then sprinkle the fruit with minced ginger and dried rosemary.

3.Bake the mango at 360F for 20 minutes.

Nutrition: 133 calories, 1.4g protein, 25.5g carbohydrates, 4.2g fat, 2.8g fiber, 0mg cholesterol, 2mg sodium, 289mg potassium

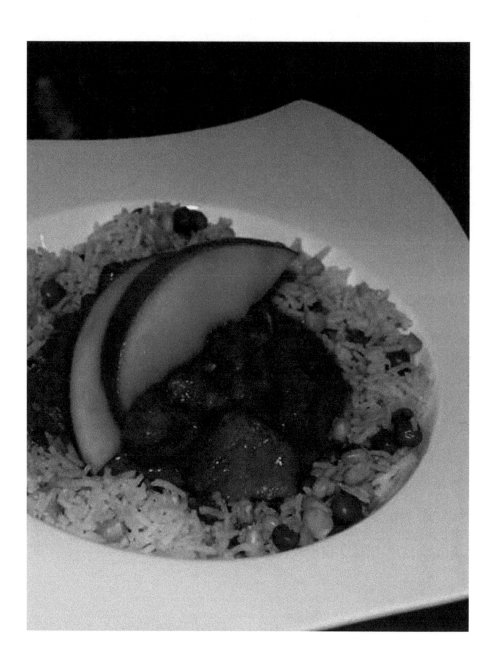

Poached Green Beans

Prep Time:
10 minutes
Cook Time:
15 minutes
Serve: 4

Ingredients:

- 1-pound green beans, trimmed
- 2 cups of water
- 1 garlic clove, diced
- 2 tablespoons olive oil
- 1 tablespoon lime juice

Directions:

1.Bring the water to boil and add green beans. Boil them for 10 minutes.

2.Then remove the green beans from water and mix with garlic clove, olive oil, and lime juice.

Nutrition: 97 calories, 2.1g protein, 8.6g carbohydrates, 7.2g fat, 3.9g fiber, 0mg cholesterol, 11mg sodium, 244mg potassium

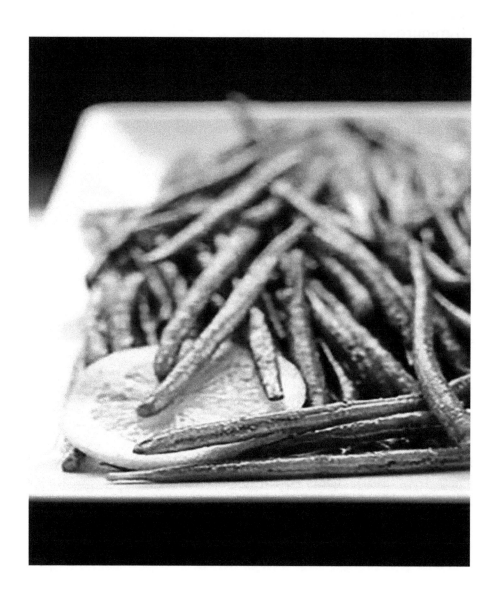